ANDREW MIRIZZI

The Newcomer's Blueprint to Health and Fitness

Build a Strong Foundation for Lasting Wellness

First edition

This book was professionally typeset on Reedsy.
Find out more at reedsy.com

"Success is the sum of small efforts, re-
peated day in and day out."

-Robert Collier

Contents

1

Introduction

Welcome to Your Journey!

Welcome to "The Newcomer's Blueprint to Health and Fitness: Build a Strong Foundation for Lasting Wellness." Whether you're just starting your health and fitness journey or looking to solidify your foundation, this book is designed to guide you every step of the way. Embarking on a path toward better health and fitness can be both exciting and daunting, but with the right tools, knowledge, and mindset, you can achieve your goals and enjoy lasting wellness.

In today's fast-paced world, maintaining a healthy lifestyle cannot be overstated. Good health and fitness are not just about looking a certain way; they are about feeling your best, both mentally and physically, and living a life full of energy and vitality. However, with the overwhelming amount of information available, it can be challenging to know where to start. This is where this book comes in.

Overview of the Book's Structure and Goals

"The Newcomer's Blueprint to Health and Fitness" is structured to provide you with a clear, step-by-step guide to building a strong foundation for your fitness journey. Here's a brief overview of what you can expect:

1. Understanding Health and Fitness: We'll begin by defining what health and fitness mean and discussing the benefits they bring to your life. This chapter will help you understand the big picture and why your efforts are worthwhile.

2. Setting Your Goals: Goal-setting is crucial for success. We'll explore how to set realistic and achievable goals that will keep you motivated and on track.

3. Nutrition Basics: A balanced diet is a cornerstone of good health. This chapter will cover the essentials of nutrition, including how to build a balanced diet and plan your meals.

4. Creating Your Fitness Plan: Designing a workout routine tailored to your needs and goals is key. We'll guide you through the process of creating a balanced fitness plan that includes different types of exercise.

5. Getting Started with Exercise: Starting a new exercise regimen can be intimidating. We'll provide tips and strategies to ease you into regular physical activity, ensuring you feel confident and prepared.

6. Staying Motivated: Maintaining motivation over the long term is often one of the biggest challenges. This chapter will offer practical strategies to keep you inspired and engaged.

7. Recovery and Rest: Rest and recovery are just as important as active

workouts. We'll discuss the best practices for allowing your body to recover and avoiding overtraining.

8. Building Healthy Habits: Sustainable changes come from healthy habits. We'll explore how to integrate fitness into your daily life and make lasting changes.

9. Special Considerations: Every individual is unique. This chapter will address how to tailor your approach based on your specific needs, health conditions, and fitness levels.

10. Creating a Support System: Having a support system can significantly impact your success. We'll discuss how to build and engage with a community that supports your goals.

Encouragement for Your Journey

Starting something new can be challenging, but remember that every expert was once a beginner. This book is here to support you, offering clear guidance, practical advice, and encouragement. Each chapter is designed to build upon the last, providing you with a comprehensive understanding and actionable steps to achieve your health and fitness goals.

As you navigate this book, remember that progress is a journey, not a destination. Celebrate your successes, no matter how small, and be kind to yourself during setbacks. Committing to improving your health and fitness is a commendable step toward a happier, healthier life.

Thank you for allowing me to be part of your journey. Let's get started on building a strong foundation for lasting wellness!

2

Chapter 2: Understanding Health and Fitness

To build a strong foundation for your wellness journey, it's essential to understand what health and fitness truly mean. This chapter explores the definitions, benefits of a healthy lifestyle, and common misconceptions that might hold you back.

Definition of Health and Fitness

Health:

Health is a state of complete physical, mental, and social well-being, not merely the absence of disease or infirmity. It encompasses everything from your physical fitness and nutritional habits to your emotional resilience and ability to connect with others.

Fitness:

Fitness refers to your body's ability to perform daily tasks efficiently, with enough energy left over for leisure and emergencies. It includes several components:

- Cardiovascular endurance: How well your heart and lungs deliver oxygen during prolonged activity.
- Muscular strength and endurance: Your muscles' ability to exert force and sustain activity over time.
- Flexibility: The range of motion of your joints and muscles.
- Body composition: The proportion of fat, muscle, bone, and other tissues in your body.

Together, health and fitness work hand-in-hand to ensure you not only look and feel good but also thrive in all areas of life.

The Benefits of a Healthy Lifestyle

Adopting a healthy lifestyle goes far beyond appearances. The benefits are holistic and impact every aspect of your life.

1. Physical Benefits:

- Increased Energy: Regular exercise and balanced nutrition provide your body with sustained energy throughout the day.
- Improved Longevity: A healthy lifestyle reduces the risk of chronic illnesses like heart disease, diabetes, and certain cancers.
- Better Sleep: Consistent activity and good nutrition promote deeper, more restorative sleep.
- Enhanced Immune Function: Proper diet, exercise, and rest strengthen your body's defense systems.

2. Mental and Emotional Benefits:

- Reduced Stress and Anxiety: Exercise releases endorphins, improving your mood and reducing stress.
- Improved Focus and Productivity: A fit body supports a sharp mind, enhancing your ability to concentrate and make decisions.
- Boosted Self-Esteem: Achieving fitness goals fosters a sense of accomplishment and confidence.

3. Social and Lifestyle Benefits:

- Stronger Relationships: Fitness activities like group classes or sports encourage social interaction and teamwork.
- Greater Independence: Maintaining strength and mobility ensures you can perform daily tasks well into old age.

Common Misconceptions About Fitness

Before diving into your fitness journey, it's important to address misconceptions that might deter or mislead you.

1. "You Need to Be Fit to Start Working Out."

- Truth: Everyone starts somewhere. Your fitness level today doesn't define your potential—it's just your starting point. Progress is made through small, consistent efforts over time.

2. "Fitness Means Looking a Certain Way."

- Truth: Fitness is about functionality, health, and feeling good in your body, not meeting a societal standard of appearance.

3. "You Have to Spend Hours at the Gym."

- Truth: Short, focused workouts can be just as effective as long sessions. What matters most is consistency and quality, not quantity.

4. "Dieting Is the Only Way to Be Healthy."

- Truth: Restrictive diets are often unsustainable. A balanced, enjoyable approach to eating is key to lasting health.

5. "Age or Medical Conditions Prevent Progress."

- Truth: Fitness is for everyone, regardless of age or health status. Exercise can be adapted to your unique needs, helping you improve mobility, strength, and overall well-being.

Putting It All Together

Understanding health and fitness is the first step toward making meaningful changes in your life. By focusing on holistic well-being and dispelling myths, you'll build a mindset that supports long-term success. Health is not a destination; it's an ongoing journey of self-care, learning, and growth.

In the next chapter, we'll explore how to set clear, actionable goals that pave the way for your personal fitness journey. Remember, this is just the beginning—every step forward is a step toward a healthier, happier you.

3

Chapter 3: Setting Your Goals

When it comes to health and fitness, having clear, defined goals is your compass. Without a destination in mind, it's easy to get lost or lose motivation. Goal-setting provides direction, focus, and a sense of accomplishment as you achieve milestones along the way. Let's dive into the importance of setting goals, how to craft effective ones using the SMART framework, and the role of tracking progress in your journey to lasting wellness.

The Importance of Goal-Setting

Think of goals as the foundation of any successful fitness plan. They help you:

- Maintain Focus: Knowing what you want to achieve prevents distractions and keeps you motivated.
- Measure Progress: Goals allow you to evaluate whether your efforts are paying off.

- Boost Confidence: Accomplishing goals, even small ones, reinforces your belief in your ability to succeed.
- Stay Committed: A well-defined goal serves as a reminder of why you started, especially during challenging times.

Without goals, workouts may feel aimless, and nutritional choices might lack direction. But when your actions are tied to a purpose, you'll notice how much easier it becomes to stay consistent and enthusiastic about your health journey.

SMART Goals: A Blueprint for Success

Not all goals are created equal. "I want to be healthier" or "I want to lose weight" may be a starting point, but they're too vague to be effective. Enter the SMART framework, a tool for creating actionable and achievable goals.

1. **S**pecific

Be clear about what you want to accomplish. Instead of saying, "I want to get fit," try something like, "I want to be able to run a 5K without stopping."

Why it matters: Specific goals give you a concrete target to aim for, making it easier to plan your actions.

2. **M**easurable

Attach metrics to your goal to track progress. For example, instead of "I want to lose weight," say, "I want to lose 10 pounds."

Why it matters: Measurable goals allow you to monitor improvements, adjust strategies, and celebrate milestones.

3. **A**chievable

Ensure your goal is realistic given your current circumstances and resources. If you're new to exercise, aiming to run a marathon in a month may not be feasible.

Why it matters: Achievable goals prevent discouragement and keep you motivated by setting you up for success.

4. **R**elevant

Your goal should align with your broader vision of health and fitness. If your priority is improving energy levels, focusing on extreme weight lifting might not be the most relevant path.

Why it matters: Relevant goals keep your efforts aligned with what truly matters to you.

5. **T**ime-bound

Set a deadline to create urgency and accountability. For instance, "I want to complete a 5K within the next three months."

Why it matters: A timeline prevents procrastination and helps you stay committed.

Short-Term vs. Long-Term Goals

To maintain momentum and perspective, it's important to balance short-term and long-term goals.

Short-Term Goals

These are milestones that can be achieved in weeks or months. Examples include:

- Completing three workouts a week for a month.
- Drinking eight glasses of water daily for 30 days.
- Reducing fast-food intake to once a week.

Short-term goals build habits and provide quick wins to keep you motivated.

Long-Term Goals

These are broader, overarching objectives that take months or years to achieve. Examples include:

- Running a marathon within a year.
- Reaching and maintaining a healthy body weight over the next 12 months.
- Building a consistent workout routine that fits into your lifestyle.

Long-term goals give your journey purpose and direction, but they're built on the foundation of consistent short-term efforts.

Tracking Your Progress

Monitoring your journey is just as important as setting goals. Progress tracking helps you stay accountable, recognize achievements, and identify areas for improvement. Here are a few ways to effectively track your progress:

1. Journaling: Record workouts, meals, energy levels, and how you're feeling overall.

2. Apps and Wearables: Use technology to monitor steps, calories, heart rate, and sleep patterns.

3. Photos and Measurements: Take pictures and body measurements at regular intervals to see changes that the scale might not capture. Some scales can measure your body fat percentage which is a great measurement because you may not be losing weight but could be losing body fat.

4. Fitness Milestones: Celebrate non-scale victories like lifting heavier weights, running faster, or mastering a new yoga pose.

Consistency in tracking doesn't just show where you've been; it illuminates the path forward.

Putting It All Together

Setting goals isn't just about envisioning an endpoint—it's about crafting a roadmap to a healthier, happier you. With SMART goals as your guide, a balance of short-term and long-term objectives, and a commitment to tracking progress, you're setting yourself up for lasting success. Take the time to define your goals today, and let them propel you toward the wellness you deserve.

4

Chapter 4: Nutrition Basics

When it comes to building a foundation for health and fitness, nutrition plays a central role. It fuels your body, aids in recovery, and supports your overall well-being. In this chapter, we'll explore the essential components of nutrition, from understanding nutrients to crafting a balanced diet. By the end, you'll have the tools to make informed food choices that align with your goals.

Understanding Macronutrients and Micronutrients

Macronutrients

Macronutrients are the primary sources of energy your body needs in large amounts. They include:

1. Carbohydrates

- Role: Your body's main energy source, particularly for physical activity and brain function.
- Sources: Whole grains, fruits, vegetables, legumes, and dairy.

Tip: Focus on complex carbs like oats, quinoa, and sweet potatoes for sustained energy.

2. Proteins

- Role: Essential for muscle repair, growth, and overall cell function.
- Sources: Lean meats, fish, eggs, tofu, beans, and dairy.

Tip: Aim for a mix of animal or plant-based proteins to diversify your diet.

3. Fats

- Role: Necessary for hormone production, brain health, and energy storage.
- Sources: Nuts, seeds, avocados, olive oil, and fatty fish like salmon.

Tip: Prioritize healthy fats over trans fats or excessive saturated fats.

Micronutrients

Micronutrients are vitamins and minerals your body needs in smaller amounts but are just as crucial for health.

- Vitamins: Support immune function, energy production, and skin health (e.g., Vitamin C, Vitamin D, and B vitamins).
- Minerals: Maintain strong bones, regulate blood pressure, and aid in muscle function (e.g., calcium, potassium, and iron).
- Sources: Found in fruits, vegetables, nuts, seeds, dairy, and lean proteins.

To ensure you're getting all the necessary micronutrients, aim for a colorful plate filled with a variety of whole foods.

The Importance of Hydration

Water is life—literally. Staying hydrated is essential for nearly every function in your body, including digestion, temperature regulation, and joint lubrication. Dehydration can lead to fatigue, reduced physical performance, and even cognitive impairment.

How Much Water Do You Need?

- A general guideline is 8–10 cups (2–2.5 liters) per day, but your needs may vary based on activity level, climate, and body size.
- During exercise, aim to drink an additional 16–20 ounces (500–600 mL) per hour of activity.

Hydration Tips:

1. Keep a reusable water bottle with you at all times.
2. Add natural flavor to your water with lemon, cucumber, or mint.
3. Include water-rich foods like cucumbers, watermelon, and oranges in your diet.
4. I highly recommend using electrolyte drops in your water as needed.
5. Although, it can be difficult try to reduce or eliminate sodas, alcohol, and coffee because they can dehydrate you. Drink more water to offset these drink's effects.

Building a Balanced Diet

A balanced diet provides the right mix of macronutrients and micronutrients for your body to function optimally. Here's how to structure your meals:

1. Half Your Plate: Vegetables and Fruits

- Prioritize a variety of colors to maximize nutrient intake.

2. A Quarter of Your Plate: Lean Proteins

- Examples include chicken, fish, tofu, eggs, or legumes.

3. A Quarter of Your Plate: Whole Grains or Starchy Veggies

- Brown rice, quinoa, sweet potatoes, or whole-grain bread are excellent choices.

4. Include Healthy Fats

- Use small amounts of nuts, seeds, avocado, or olive oil for flavor and satiety.

5. Limit Added Sugars and Processed Foods

- Treat them as occasional indulgences, not daily staples.

Meal Planning and Prep for Beginners

Meal planning and preparation can save time, reduce stress, and help you make healthier choices. Here's how to get started:

1. Plan Your Week

   - Choose recipes and snacks for the week, and make a shopping list.
   - Balance variety with consistency—rotate favorite meals but try one new recipe weekly.

2. Prep Ahead

   - Wash and chop vegetables for salads or stir-fries.
   - Cook grains and proteins in bulk to use throughout the week.

3. Invest in Storage

   - Use airtight containers to portion meals and keep ingredients fresh.

4. Batch Cooking

   - Prepare soups, casseroles, or slow-cooker meals that can be refrigerated or frozen.

Sample Meal Prep Plan:

- Breakfast: Overnight oats with berries and almond butter.
- Lunch: Grilled chicken, quinoa, and roasted vegetables.
- Snack: Greek yogurt with a handful of nuts.
- Dinner: Stir-fried tofu, brown rice, and steamed broccoli.

Healthy Snack Options

Snacks can be part of a balanced diet when chosen wisely. Opt for nutrient-dense options that provide sustained energy:

- Fresh Fruits and Nuts: A handful of almonds with an apple.
- Vegetables with Hummus: Carrot sticks, cucumber slices, or bell peppers.
- Greek Yogurt with Berries: High in protein and antioxidants.
- Rice Cakes with Nut Butter: A light but satisfying option.
- Hard-Boiled Eggs: Easy to prepare and portable.
- Homemade Energy Bars: Use oats, peanut butter, and a touch of honey.

Putting It All Together

Mastering the basics of nutrition doesn't mean striving for perfection—it's about making small, consistent choices that add up over time. By understanding macronutrients and micronutrients, staying hydrated, building balanced meals, and planning ahead, you'll create a sustainable approach to eating. Start with one or two changes this week, and watch how they transform your energy, mood, and performance. Healthy eating is a skill, and with practice, it will become second nature and become your lifestyle.

5

Chapter 5: Creating Your Fitness Plan

Creating a fitness plan is like building a roadmap to your goals. It ensures you're exercising efficiently, safely, and in alignment with your unique needs. This chapter will guide you through assessing your current fitness level, exploring different types of exercise, designing a balanced workout routine, and progressively increasing intensity to achieve lasting results.

Assessing Your Current Fitness Level

Before diving into a workout routine, it's important to understand where you're starting from. Assessing your fitness level helps you set realistic goals and tailor your plan to suit your abilities. Here's how to do it:

1. Evaluate Your Cardiovascular Endurance

- Test Idea: Walk or jog for 1 mile and record how long it takes and how you feel afterward.
- Purpose: Provides a baseline for your heart and lung fitness.

2. Measure Strength

- Test Idea: Count how many push-ups, squats, or sit-ups you can perform in one minute.
- Purpose: Gauges your muscular endurance and strength.

3. Check Flexibility

- Test Idea: Perform a sit-and-reach test by sitting on the floor with legs extended and reaching forward as far as possible.
- Purpose: Assesses the flexibility of your lower back and hamstrings.

4. Assess Balance

- Test Idea: Stand on one foot for as long as possible. Repeat on the other side.
- Purpose: Determines your balance and stability.

Write down your results to establish a baseline and use them to track your progress over time.

Types of Exercise: Cardio, Strength Training, Flexibility, and Balance

Incorporating a variety of exercise types into your routine ensures comprehensive fitness. Each type serves a unique purpose:

1. Cardiovascular Exercise (Cardio)

- Benefits: Improves heart health, burns calories, and boosts endurance.
- Examples: Running, cycling, swimming, brisk walking, or dance-based workouts.

Tip: Start with moderate-intensity sessions (e.g., 20–30 minutes) and gradually increase duration.

2. Strength Training

- Benefits: Builds muscle, increases metabolism, and improves bone density.
- Examples: Weightlifting, resistance bands, bodyweight exercises like push-ups and squats.

Tip: Aim for 2–3 sessions per week, targeting all major muscle groups.

3. Flexibility Training

- Benefits: Enhances range of motion, reduces injury risk, and improves posture.
- Examples: Yoga, Pilates, dynamic stretches, or static stretches after workouts.

Tip: Spend at least 5–10 minutes stretching daily or after exercise.

4. Balance Training

- Benefits: Improves stability, and coordination and reduces fall risk (especially important as you age).
- Examples: Standing on one leg, tai chi, stability ball exercises.

Tip: Incorporate balance exercises 2–3 times a week.

Designing a Balanced Workout Routine

A well-rounded fitness plan incorporates all four types of exercise, tailored to your goals and fitness level. Here's an example for beginners:

Weekly Workout Plan:

Day	Activity
Monday	30 minutes brisk walking (cardio) + 5 minutes stretching
Tuesday	Full-body strength workout (e.g., bodyweight exercises)
Wednesday	Yoga or Pilates (flexibility and balance)
Thursday	20–25 minutes cycling or swimming (cardio)
Friday	Strength workout: focus on upper or lower body
Saturday	Hike or fun physical activity of choice (active recovery)
Sunday	Rest or gentle stretching

Tips for Success:

1. Start with shorter workouts and gradually build up duration.
2. Alternate between high-intensity and low-intensity days to allow recovery.
3. Listen to your body—rest if you feel overly fatigued or sore.

How to Gradually Increase Intensity

Progressing your fitness routine is key to improving strength, endurance, and flexibility. However, it's important to increase intensity safely and sustainably.

1. The Principle of Progressive Overload

To see results, you must gradually challenge your body by increasing the demand placed on it. This can be done by:

- Cardio: Increase the speed, duration, or incline of your sessions.
- Strength: Add more weight, reps, or sets to your exercises.
- Flexibility: Hold stretches longer or try advanced poses.

2. The 10% Rule

Avoid injury by making small adjustments. For example, increase your running distance or weightlifting volume by no more than 10% per week.

3. Monitor Your Recovery

Ensure your body is adapting well by tracking how you feel after workouts. Signs you're progressing too quickly include persistent fatigue, pain, or a plateau in performance.

4. Mix It Up

Prevent boredom and plateaus by varying exercises, intensities, and formats. For instance, alternate between steady-state cardio and interval training, or try new strength training exercises.

Putting It All Together

Creating your fitness plan is about finding what works for you and staying consistent. Start by assessing your fitness level, incorporate a mix of exercise types, and follow a structured routine. Most importantly, focus on gradual progress—small, sustainable changes lead to long-term success. Remember, your fitness plan is flexible and can evolve as you grow stronger and more confident. Take the first step today, and you'll be amazed at what you can achieve.

6

Chapter 6: Getting Started with Exercise

Beginning an exercise routine can feel both exciting and overwhelming. The key to success is starting where you are, addressing common challenges, and finding activities that resonate with you. This chapter will provide practical tips for beginners, guide you in choosing the right workout environment, explain workout gear essentials, and help you discover activities that make fitness enjoyable.

Tips for Beginners: Overcoming Barriers to Entry

Starting an exercise routine comes with challenges, but most barriers can be overcome with a bit of planning and a positive mindset.

1. Address Common Barriers

• "I don't have time."

Solution: Schedule short workouts (15–30 minutes) and treat them like appointments. Even small sessions add up over time.

- "I don't know where to start."

Solution: Begin with simple activities like walking, stretching, or bodyweight exercises. Apps, videos, or beginner classes can also help.

- "I'm not motivated."

Solution: Focus on your "why". Is it better health, more energy, or improving your confidence? Start small, and momentum will build.

- "I'm too self-conscious."

Solution: Remember, everyone starts somewhere. Choose a comfortable environment, like home workouts or a supportive gym.

2. Start Small and Build Gradually

- Begin with just two or three sessions per week and increase as you feel ready.
- Focus on consistency rather than intensity—it's better to do moderate workouts regularly than to overdo it and burn out.

3. Celebrate Small Wins

- Acknowledge every step forward, from completing your first workout to trying a new exercise. These small victories add up to big results.

How to Choose the Right Gym or Workout Environment

Your workout environment plays a significant role in maintaining motivation and consistency. Whether it's a gym, studio, or outdoor space, finding the right fit is essential.

Factors to Consider:

1. Convenience: Choose a location close to your home or workplace to reduce excuses.

2. Atmosphere:

- If you enjoy community, opt for group classes or gyms with a welcoming vibe.
- If you prefer solitude, home workouts or quieter gym hours may suit you better.

3. Equipment and Services:

- Look for facilities that match your needs, such as free weights, machines, yoga mats, or swimming pools.

4. Budget:

- Compare options like gym memberships, pay-per-class studios, or free outdoor spaces to find what fits your budget.

5. Trial Periods:

- Many gyms offer free trials. Use these to assess whether the environment feels comfortable and supportive.

At-Home Options:

If going to a gym doesn't appeal to you, at-home workouts are highly effective. You can use minimal equipment like resistance bands, dumbbells, or even your own body weight. Online videos and apps provide guidance and variety.

Understanding Workout Gear and Equipment Essentials

Having the right gear can make your workouts more comfortable and enjoyable. Here's what you'll need to get started:

Clothing:

- Breathable fabrics: Choose moisture-wicking materials to stay cool and dry.
- Proper fit: Ensure your clothes allow freedom of movement without being too loose or restrictive.

Footwear:

Select shoes that match your activity. For example:

- Running shoes for cardio.
- Cross-trainers for gym workouts.
- Court shoes for sports like basketball or tennis.
- Visit a specialty store to get fitted if you're unsure.

Basic Equipment for Beginners:

- Yoga Mat: Great for stretching, yoga, and bodyweight exercises.

- Resistance Bands: Versatile and easy to store, perfect for strength training.
- Dumbbells: Start with light weights (2–10 lbs) and increase as you gain strength.
- Water Bottle: Staying hydrated is essential during any workout.

Optional Extras:

- A fitness tracker or smartwatch to monitor your progress.
- Foam roller for post-workout recovery and muscle soreness relief.

Finding Fun Activities You Enjoy

The best exercise is the one you'll stick with. Enjoyment is key to staying consistent and making fitness a long-term habit.

Explore Different Options:
1. Team Sports: Basketball, soccer, or volleyball for those who enjoy camaraderie and competition.
2. Dance Classes: Zumba, hip-hop, or ballroom for a fun and rhythmic way to stay active.
3. Outdoor Adventures: Hiking, cycling, or kayaking to connect with nature while exercising.
4. Group Classes: Yoga, Pilates, spin, or boot camps for variety and community.
5. At-Home Workouts: Follow along with YouTube videos or fitness apps tailored to your preferences.

Experiment Until You Find Your Fit:

- Try one new activity each week. If it doesn't resonate, move on to something else.
- Invite friends or family to join you—it can make trying new activities less intimidating and more enjoyable.

Make Fitness Part of Your Lifestyle:

- Incorporate movement into daily life, like walking to work, gardening, or playing with kids.
- Remember, exercise doesn't always have to feel like a chore.

Putting It All Together

Getting started with exercise is a journey that begins with small, manageable steps. Overcoming barriers, choosing the right environment, and having the proper gear can make a significant difference. Most importantly, focus on finding activities that bring you joy—fitness is about creating a healthier, happier life, and enjoyment is the cornerstone of sustainability. Start today, and let the fun of movement guide your path to wellness.

7

Chapter 7: Staying Motivated

Embarking on a health and fitness journey is one thing; staying committed is another. Motivation can ebb and flow, but with the right strategies, you can maintain consistency and overcome challenges. In this chapter, we'll explore how to stay motivated, the importance of accountability, celebrating progress, and managing setbacks with resilience.

Strategies to Maintain Motivation

Motivation isn't something you can always rely on—it fluctuates based on mood, energy, and circumstances. The key is to create systems and habits that keep you moving forward even on less-motivated days.

1. Set Clear and Meaningful Goals

- Revisit your goals often to remind yourself of "why" you started.
- Keep them specific and personally significant, like improving energy to play with your kids or gaining confidence to try new activities.

2. Focus on Habits, Not Just Results

- Create a routine by scheduling workouts at the same time each day.
- Pair your workouts with something enjoyable, like listening to music or a favorite podcast.

3. Use Visual Reminders

- Keep a calendar where you mark completed workouts. Seeing progress builds momentum.
- Post inspiring quotes or pictures in your workout space to stay focused.

4. Change It Up

- Avoid monotony by trying new activities, exploring different workout formats, or challenging yourself with fresh goals.
- Rotate between cardio, strength training, yoga, or outdoor sports to keep things interesting.

5. Reward Yourself

- Treat yourself to non-food rewards like new workout gear, a massage, or a fun outing after reaching a milestone.

The Role of Accountability: Finding a Workout Buddy or Coach

Accountability can be a powerful motivator. Sharing your goals with others and working together creates a sense of responsibility and encouragement.

Workout Buddy

- Exercising with a friend can make workouts more enjoyable and less intimidating.
- You're less likely to skip sessions when someone is counting on you.

Join a Community

- Look for group fitness classes, local running clubs, or online fitness forums to connect with like-minded individuals.
- Being part of a community fosters camaraderie and mutual encouragement.

Hire a Coach or Trainer

- A professional can provide expertise, personalized plans, and motivation.
- Trainers can help you overcome plateaus and ensure proper technique for safety and efficiency.

Digital Accountability

- Use apps or trackers to log workouts and progress.
- Share milestones on social media or fitness groups to receive support

and encouragement.

Celebrating Milestones and Achievements

Acknowledging progress, no matter how small, reinforces your efforts and keeps you motivated.

Track Your Wins

- Keep a fitness journal to note improvements, such as increased strength, endurance, or flexibility.
- Document non-scale victories like improved mood, better sleep, or fitting into old clothes.

Set Incremental Goals

- Break long-term goals into smaller, manageable milestones.
- Celebrate achievements like completing a month of consistent workouts or running your first mile without stopping.

Make Celebrations Special

- Reward yourself with experiences, such as a hike in a new location or attending a fun dance class.
- Reflect on your journey and appreciate how far you've come.

Dealing with Setbacks and Obstacles

Setbacks are inevitable, but they don't have to derail your progress. The key is to approach them with a growth mindset.

1. Reframe Challenges

- View setbacks as learning opportunities rather than failures.
- Ask yourself, "What can I do differently next time?"

2. Practice Self-Compassion

- Be kind to yourself during tough times.
- Remember, progress isn't linear—it's okay to have off days or weeks. Don't beat yourself up!

3. Identify the Cause

- Reflect on what led to the setback (e.g., lack of time, stress, or unrealistic expectations).
- Adjust your approach to address these barriers.

4. Get Back on Track

- Start small if you've taken a break—resume with lighter workouts or shorter sessions.
- Reconnect with your goals and remind yourself of why they matter.

5. Seek Support

- Lean on friends, family, or a fitness community to help you through challenging periods.
- A coach or therapist can also provide guidance if motivation feels out of reach.

Putting It All Together

Staying motivated is about consistency, adaptability, and celebrating your journey. By setting clear goals, leaning on accountability, and embracing challenges as part of the process, you'll create a sustainable approach to health and fitness. Remember, motivation may waver, but discipline and the support of others will carry you through. Every step forward, no matter how small, is a victory. Stay committed, stay kind to yourself, and most importantly, enjoy the process.

8

Chapter 8: Recovery and Rest

Fitness isn't just about the time spent exercising—it's also about how effectively you recover. Recovery and rest are critical for allowing your body to rebuild, grow stronger, and avoid injury. In this chapter, we'll discuss why rest days are essential, explore recovery techniques, examine the role of sleep in fitness, and help you recognize the signs of overtraining.

The Importance of Rest Days

Rest days aren't a sign of slacking—they're an integral part of any fitness routine.

Why Rest Days Matter:
1. Muscle Repair and Growth:

- Exercise creates tiny tears in your muscles, which heal during rest, making them stronger.

2. Injury Prevention:

- Overuse without rest increases the risk of strains, sprains, or burnout.

3. Improved Performance:

- Rest days replenish energy stores (glycogen) and help you perform better in future workouts.

4. Mental Rejuvenation:

- Taking a break can reduce stress and improve motivation to stick with your routine.

How Often Should You Rest?

- For most people, one to two rest days per week is ideal.
- Active rest days, such as gentle yoga or a leisurely walk, can help you stay active without overexerting.

Techniques for Recovery: Stretching, Foam Rolling, and More

Active recovery techniques can enhance the body's healing process and reduce soreness.

1. Stretching

- Benefits: Improves flexibility, increases blood flow, and helps relax tight muscles.

When to Stretch:

- Dynamic stretches before workouts to warm up.
- Static stretches after workouts to release tension.

2. Foam Rolling (Self-Myofascial Release)

- Benefits: Relieves muscle tightness, reduces soreness, and improves circulation.

How to Use a Foam Roller:

- Slowly roll over sore or tight muscles, pausing on tender spots for 20–30 seconds.
- Focus on areas like your thighs, calves, back, and shoulders.

3. Massage Therapy

- Professional massages can alleviate deep muscle tension and improve relaxation.
- Consider incorporating self-massage tools, like massage balls or handheld devices, for convenience.

4. Hydration and Nutrition

- Drink water and consume a balanced post-workout meal with protein and carbohydrates to aid recovery.
- Foods rich in antioxidants (e.g., berries, and spinach) can help reduce inflammation.

5. Cold and Heat Therapy

- Cold Therapy: Ice baths or cold packs can reduce inflammation and soreness after intense workouts.
- Heat Therapy: Heating pads or warm baths promote relaxation and increase blood flow to aid recovery.

Understanding Sleep's Role in Fitness

Sleep is often overlooked but is a cornerstone of effective recovery.

How Sleep Impacts Fitness:
1. Muscle Repair:

- Growth hormone, crucial for muscle repair, is released during deep sleep.

2. Energy Restoration:

- Sleep restores energy reserves and prepares your body for the next day's activities.

3. Mental Focus:

- Quality sleep improves focus and reaction time, essential for safe and effective workouts.

4. Weight Management:

- Sleep helps regulate hunger hormones, reducing cravings and supporting healthy eating habits.

Tips for Better Sleep:

- Aim for 7–9 hours of sleep per night.
- Establish a bedtime routine, such as reading or meditating, to signal your body that it's time to wind down.
- Limit caffeine and screen time in the hours leading up to bedtime.

Listening to Your Body: Signs of Overtraining

Overtraining can derail your progress and lead to burnout or injury. It's crucial to recognize when your body needs more rest.

Common Signs of Overtraining:
1. Persistent Fatigue:

- Feeling drained even after a good night's sleep.

2. Decreased Performance:

- Struggling to lift weights or complete workouts that were previously manageable.

3. Mood Changes:

- Irritability, anxiety, or lack of motivation.

4. Physical Symptoms:

- Increased soreness, frequent injuries, or recurring colds.

5. Sleep Issues:

- Difficulty falling or staying asleep.

What to Do if You're Overtraining:

- Take an extended rest period, ranging from a few days to a week, to allow your body to recover.
- Adjust your workout intensity or volume when you resume exercising.
- Incorporate regular rest days and recovery practices into your routine moving forward.

Putting It All Together

Recovery is just as important as the effort you put into your workouts. By embracing rest days, using recovery techniques, prioritizing sleep, and paying attention to your body's signals, you can avoid burnout and stay on track toward your goals. Remember, rest and recovery aren't setbacks—they're stepping stones to better performance, greater strength, and lasting wellness. Take the time your body needs, and it will reward you with progress and resilience.

9

Chapter 9: Building Healthy Habits

Achieving lasting fitness and wellness goes beyond short-term goals. It's about building habits that become a natural part of your daily life. This chapter explores how to integrate fitness into your routine, create sustainable lifestyle changes, harness the power of consistency, and prioritize mental well-being through mindfulness.

Tips for Integrating Fitness into Daily Life

For fitness to become a habit, it must fit seamlessly into your existing lifestyle.

1. Start Small

- Begin with manageable changes, such as a 10-minute walk or a short stretching session.
- Gradually build on these habits as they become second nature.

2. Plan Ahead

- Schedule workouts like appointments. Treat them as non-negotiable.
- Pack a gym bag the night before or set up your workout space at home to eliminate excuses.

3. Combine Fitness with Daily Tasks

- Walk or bike to work if possible.
- Do squats or lunges while waiting for food to cook or watching TV.
- Take the stairs instead of the elevator.

4. Make It Social

- Invite friends or family to join you for a workout or a hike.
- Participate in group classes or local fitness events to build camaraderie.

5. Embrace Variety

- Keep things interesting by rotating activities: strength training one day, yoga the next, and a dance class later in the week.

Making Sustainable Lifestyle Changes

Sustainability is key to long-term success. Avoid drastic changes that are hard to maintain, and focus on gradual improvements.

1. Shift Your Mindset

- View fitness and wellness as a lifelong journey, not a temporary fix.
- Focus on how you feel rather than just external results, like weight or appearance.

2. Balance is Everything

- Aim for a mix of exercise, healthy eating, rest, and enjoyment.
- Allow yourself occasional indulgences without guilt—wellness is about balance, not perfection.

3. Build on Existing Habits

- Anchor new habits to ones you already do.

For example:

- Stretch after brushing your teeth in the morning.
- Do a short workout while your coffee brews.

4. Track Your Progress

- Use a journal or app to monitor your fitness activities, nutrition, and how you're feeling overall.

- Regular tracking helps you stay accountable and identify what's working.

The Power of Routine and Consistency

Consistency is the foundation of habit formation. Creating a routine simplifies decision-making and builds momentum.

1. Create a Fitness Routine

- Choose a consistent time for exercise, whether it's early morning, during lunch, or after work.
- Keep your routine flexible enough to adjust if your schedule changes but structured enough to provide stability.

2. Celebrate the Process

- Focus on showing up, even if the workout isn't perfect. The act of maintaining consistency is a victory.
- Over time, consistency compounds, leading to noticeable progress.

3. Use Habit Stacking

- Pair fitness activities with everyday routines:
- Meditate for 5 minutes after your workout.
- Do a quick warm-up before starting your workday.

4. Build Resilience

- Missing a workout occasionally is normal. Instead of giving up, get back on track the next day.
- Remember: Progress is built over time, not through perfection.

Mindfulness and Mental Health in Fitness

Fitness isn't just about physical health—it's deeply connected to mental well-being. Incorporating mindfulness can make your journey more fulfilling and sustainable.

1. Be Present in Your Workouts

- Focus on how your body feels as you move. This improves performance and reduces the risk of injury.
- Pay attention to your breathing, posture, and muscle engagement.

2. Use Exercise as a Stress-Relief Tool

- Physical activity releases endorphins, which boost mood and reduce stress.
- Activities like yoga, tai chi, or a simple walk can calm the mind and promote relaxation.

3. Practice Gratitude

- Reflect on what your body can do rather than focusing on perceived limitations.

- Celebrate the effort you put into improving your health, no matter how small.

4. Balance Rest and Activity

- Avoid overtraining, as it can lead to mental fatigue and burnout.
- Incorporate activities that rejuvenate both your body and mind, like stretching or nature walks.

Putting It All Together

Building healthy habits is a gradual process that requires intention, patience, and consistency. By integrating fitness into your daily life, making sustainable lifestyle changes, and prioritizing mental well-being, you'll create a foundation for lasting wellness. Remember, habits aren't built overnight, but with time and persistence, they become second nature. Celebrate your progress, trust the process, and enjoy the journey to a healthier, happier you.

10

Chapter 10: Special Considerations

Fitness isn't one-size-fits-all. Everyone's journey is unique and influenced by individual fitness levels, health conditions, and personal goals. This chapter focuses on how to adapt to exercises to suit your needs, considerations for exercising with health conditions, and the benefits of seeking professional guidance to ensure safe and effective progress.

Modifying Exercises for Different Fitness Levels

Whether you're a beginner or more advanced, it's important to tailor exercises to match your abilities and gradually increase intensity as you progress.

1. Start Where You Are
   Beginners:

- Focus on mastering basic movements with proper form before adding intensity.

- Opt for bodyweight exercises like squats, push-ups (on knees if needed), and planks.

Intermediate:

- Incorporate weights or resistance bands to build strength and add variety.
- Try compound movements like lunges with bicep curls or weighted squats.

Advanced:

- Increase intensity with heavier weights, advanced variations (e.g., single-leg squats), or high-intensity interval training (HIIT).

2. Listen to Your Body

- Modify workouts to avoid pain or discomfort. Discomfort may indicate a need to adjust form, reduce weight, or scale back intensity.
- If an exercise feels too easy, increase repetitions, resistance, or duration to challenge yourself.

3. Use Progression Plans

- Gradually increase the difficulty by following structured plans that align with your goals, such as Couch-to-5K for running or beginner-to-intermediate weightlifting programs.

4. Incorporate Adaptive Options

- Swap high-impact exercises for low-impact alternatives when needed. For example, replace jumping jacks with step jacks or burpees with incline push-ups.

Health Conditions and Fitness: What to Consider

Your health history and any existing conditions should guide your approach to fitness. Exercise can benefit most conditions, but it's essential to prioritize safety.

1. Talk to Your Doctor

- Before starting a new fitness program, especially if you have chronic conditions (e.g., diabetes, heart disease, arthritis), consult your healthcare provider.
- Get clearance and specific recommendations tailored to your condition.

2. Exercise Modifications for Common Conditions

- Joint Pain/Arthritis:
- Focus on low-impact activities like swimming, cycling, or yoga.
- Include gentle strength training to support joint health.

Cardiovascular Conditions:

- Begin with light to moderate intensity exercises such as walking or

stationary biking.
- Monitor heart rate and avoid sudden spikes in exertion.

Diabetes:

- Include a mix of cardio and strength training to improve insulin sensitivity.
- Check blood sugar levels before and after exercise and have a snack on hand if needed.

Pregnancy:

- Opt for low-impact activities like prenatal yoga, swimming, or walking.
- Avoid exercises that require lying flat on your back after the first trimester or those with a high risk of falling.

3. Recognize Warning Signs
Stop exercising immediately if you experience:

- Chest pain or tightness.
- Shortness of breath not typical for exercise.
- Dizziness or nausea.
- Unusual joint pain or swelling.

Working with Professionals: Trainers, Nutritionists, and Doctors

Partnering with professionals can provide valuable guidance and support, especially if you're new to fitness, have specific goals, or face health challenges.

1. Personal Trainers

When to Hire a Trainer:

- If you're unsure how to start or want personalized plans to reach your goals.
- To ensure proper form and technique, reducing the risk of injury.

What to Look For:

- Certifications from reputable organizations (e.g., ACE, NASM, ACSM).
- Experience in working with clients of your fitness level or with specific conditions.

2. Nutritionists or Dietitians

When to Consult a Nutrition Expert:

- To create a nutrition plan tailored to your goals (e.g., weight loss, muscle gain).
- If you have dietary restrictions or health concerns (e.g., allergies, IBS).

Credentials to Check:

- Registered Dietitian (RD) or equivalent certifications.
- Specializations in sports nutrition or clinical nutrition, if applicable.

3. Medical Professionals
When to Seek Medical Advice:

- If you're recovering from an injury or surgery.
- When managing chronic conditions that affect mobility, energy levels, or safety during exercise.

Working with Physical Therapists:

- For targeted exercises to address injuries, improve mobility, or prevent re-injury.

Putting It All Together

Special considerations make your fitness journey uniquely yours. By modifying exercises, taking health conditions into account, and collaborating with professionals, you can create a safe, effective, and sustainable approach to wellness. Remember, there's no "one-size-fits-all" in fitness—success lies in finding what works best for your body, needs, and lifestyle. Embrace your individuality, listen to your body, and don't hesitate to seek guidance to achieve your goals safely and confidently.

11

Chapter 11: Creating a Support System

No fitness journey happens in isolation. Building a support system is essential for maintaining motivation, overcoming challenges, and celebrating successes. In this chapter, we'll explore why community matters, how to find both online and local fitness resources, and ways to share your journey with the people who matter most.

The Importance of Community and Support

A strong support system provides encouragement, accountability, and a sense of belonging, all of which are vital for long-term success.

1. Why Support Matters:
   Motivation Boost:

   - Surrounding yourself with like-minded individuals keeps you inspired and focused on your goals.

Accountability:

- Having someone to check in with makes you less likely to skip workouts or stray from your plan.

Shared Experiences:

- Connecting with others on a similar journey reminds you that you're not alone and that challenges are normal.

Emotional Support:

- Fitness ups and downs can be easier to handle when someone is cheering you on or offering encouragement.

2. The Role of Positive Influence:

- Surround yourself with people who support your goals rather than those who might unintentionally discourage you.

Finding Online Resources and Communities

In the digital age, online platforms offer endless opportunities to connect with others and learn from their experiences.

1. Social Media Groups and Forums

- Join fitness-focused communities on platforms like Facebook, Reddit, or specialized apps like Strava or MyFitnessPal.

- Look for groups aligned with your interests, such as beginners' fitness, weightlifting, or yoga enthusiasts.

2. Fitness Apps and Virtual Classes

- Many apps not only track progress, but also have community features where you can share milestones or compete in friendly challenges.
- Virtual classes often include chat features, allowing participants to connect and motivate one another.

3. Inspirational Content

- Follow fitness influencers, bloggers, or YouTubers who align with your values and goals.
- Use their content for tips, and encouragement to see how others navigate their fitness journeys.

4. Be Cautious Online

- Not all advice or groups are helpful—prioritize supportive communities and credible sources.
- Avoid comparison traps; everyone's journey is unique.

Engaging with Local Fitness Groups or Classes

In-person connections can offer a sense of camaraderie and provide opportunities to make fitness fun and social.

1. Benefits of Local Groups:
   Real-Time Interaction:

   - Face-to-face support builds trust and friendships that can extend beyond workouts.

Guided Expertise:

   - Instructors or group leaders often provide structured, safe workouts.

Accountability:

   - Knowing others expect you to show up can help you stick to your routine.

2. Where to Find Local Fitness Groups:

   - Check community centers, gyms, or local parks for group fitness classes like Zumba, Pilates, or running clubs.
   - Explore meetups for outdoor activities like hiking, cycling, or even recreational sports leagues.

3. Volunteering Through Fitness:

   - Join charity events such as 5Ks or fitness fundraisers to meet like-minded people while supporting a cause.

Sharing Your Journey with Friends and Family

Your closest relationships can play a significant role in your fitness journey.

1. Involve Your Inner Circle:
   Invite Participation:

   - Ask a friend or family member to join you for workouts, hikes, or fitness challenges.

Share Your Goals:

   - Let them know what you're working toward and how they can support you.

2. Lead by Example:

   - Inspire others by showing how your fitness journey improves your overall well-being.
   - Avoid pressuring anyone; focus on sharing your positive experiences.

3. Overcoming Resistance:

   - Some people may not understand or support your new habits initially.
   - Be patient and explain how these changes benefit your health and happiness.

4. Celebrate Together:

- Include loved ones in celebrating milestones, whether it's a new personal best or completing a fitness program.
- Acknowledging small victories fosters a sense of shared accomplishment.

Putting It All Together

Fitness is not just a solo endeavor—it's a communal experience that thrives on connection. By building a robust support system, both online and in person, you'll stay motivated, feel accountable, and enjoy the journey more fully. Whether you find your tribe at the gym, in a virtual space, or among your friends and family, the encouragement and camaraderie they offer can make all the difference. So, reach out, connect, and let others be part of your path to wellness. Together, you're stronger.

12

Chapter 12: Conclusion: Your Blueprint for a Lifetime of Wellness

Congratulations on taking the first steps toward a healthier, stronger, and more vibrant you! This journey isn't about perfection but about consistent effort, growth, and learning. As you continue on this path, let's recap the key lessons, offer encouragement for the road ahead, and provide resources to deepen your understanding and sustain your progress.

Recap of Key Points

1. Set Clear Goals:

- Start with SMART goals—Specific, Measurable, Achievable, Relevant, and Time-bound—to give your journey structure and purpose.
- Balance short-term achievements with long-term aspirations.

2. Understand the Basics:

- Nutrition is a cornerstone of fitness; focus on balanced meals, hydration, and mindful eating.
- Exercise includes a variety of components—cardio, strength, flexibility, and balance—all of which are essential for a well-rounded routine.

3. Build Sustainable Habits:

- Consistency and routine are the foundation of lasting wellness.
- Start small, make gradual changes, and embrace a mindset of lifelong growth.

4. Adapt to Your Needs:

- Modify exercises to fit your fitness level, health conditions, and personal preferences.
- Listen to your body, prioritize recovery, and seek professional guidance when necessary.

5. Create a Support System:

- Surround yourself with people who encourage and inspire you, both online and in person.
- Share your journey with friends and family, and celebrate milestones together.

Encouragement for Continued Growth and Learning

Your fitness journey is unique, and it's yours to shape. Remember that progress isn't always linear—there will be ups and downs, but every step forward, no matter how small, brings you closer to your goals.

Stay Curious:

- Continue exploring new workouts, recipes, and techniques. Variety keeps things exciting and prevents plateaus.

Be Patient:

- Fitness is a lifelong journey, not a race. Celebrate incremental progress and remain resilient through challenges.

Focus on Wellness Beyond Fitness:

- Mental health, mindfulness, and self-care are just as important as physical fitness.

You've built a foundation—now, it's time to keep building. Trust in your ability to grow stronger, healthier, and more confident with every step.

13

Chapter 13: Resources for Further Reading and Exploration

To deepen your understanding and stay inspired, here are some recommended resources:

Books:

- **Atomic Habits** by James Clear – A guide to building habits that stick.
- **The New Rules of Lifting** by Lou Schuler and Alwyn Cosgrove – A practical resource for strength training.
- **Intuitive Eating** by Evelyn Tribole and Elyse Resch – A fresh approach to building a healthy relationship with food.

Podcasts:

- **The Model Health Show** – Discussions on fitness, nutrition, and overall wellness.
- **FoundMyFitness** with Dr. Rhonda Patrick – Insights into the science

behind health and fitness.

- **Hurdle** – Stories of how people overcome obstacles through fitness and wellness.

Apps:

- **MyFitnessPal**: For tracking nutrition and exercise.
- **Couch to 5K**: A great starting point for beginner runners.
- **Yoga with Adriene** (YouTube): Accessible yoga classes for all levels.

Communities and Websites:

- Local gym or fitness studio websites often feature class schedules and events.
- Online forums like Reddit's **r/Fitness** or **r/ProgressPics** provide support and inspiration.
- Fitness blogs or social media accounts from certified professionals.

Your Next Steps

Now it's time to apply what you've learned. Start by reviewing your goals, creating a plan, and taking action. Embrace the process, stay consistent, and remind yourself why you started.

You have all the tools you need to thrive. The journey to fitness and wellness is an ongoing adventure—one filled with opportunities to grow stronger, learn more, and inspire others. Keep moving forward, and remember, every small step counts.

Here's to a lifetime of health, happiness, and fulfillment!

Invitation to Share Your Experience

Thank you for taking the time to explore *The Newcomer's Blueprint to Health and Fitness*. I hope you've found valuable insights to start or continue your fitness journey. If you've enjoyed the book and found it helpful, please consider leaving a review on Amazon. Your feedback not only helps me improve but also inspires others who are looking for guidance and motivation.

Thank you for being part of this fitness community, and I wish you success on your path to lasting wellness!

14

Chapter 14: Appendices

The following appendices provide additional tools, examples, and resources to help you apply the concepts from this book and continue your fitness and wellness journey.

Appendix A: Sample Workout Plans for Beginners

1. Weekly Full-Body Workout Plan
   Goal: Build strength, endurance, and flexibility.

Day	Activity	Duration	Notes
Monday	Cardio: Brisk walking or cycling	20–30 min	Moderate intensity
Tuesday	Strength: Bodyweight exercises	30 min	Squats, push-ups, planks, lunges
Wednesday	Flexibility: Yoga or stretching routine	20 min	Focus on breath and relaxation
Thursday	Cardio: Intervals (e.g., walk/jog mix)	20–25 min	Alternate 1 min fast, 2 min slow
Friday	Strength: Resistance bands or weights	30 min	Rows, deadlifts, shoulder presses
Saturday	Active rest: Light activities	15–20 min	Play a sport, hike, or leisure walk
Sunday	Rest or gentle stretching	–	Recovery focus

Appendix B: Sample Meal Plans and Recipes

1. One-Day Balanced Meal Plan
   Goal: Provide balanced macronutrients and essential nutrients.

Meal	Food Ideas	Notes
Breakfast	Oatmeal with fresh fruit and nuts	Add chia seeds or flax for fiber
Snack	Greek yogurt with honey and granola	High in protein
Lunch	Grilled chicken salad with olive oil	Include leafy greens, avocado
Snack	Veggie sticks with hummus	Carrots, celery, or cucumber
Dinner	Baked salmon, quinoa, and steamed broccoli	Add lemon for flavor

2. Recipe: Quick Protein Smoothie
   Ingredients:

- 1 cup almond milk
- 1 banana
- 1 scoop protein powder (optional)
- 1 tablespoon peanut butter
- Ice cubes

Instructions: Blend all ingredients until smooth. Perfect for a post-workout snack.

Appendix C: Recommended Resources

Books

- **You Are Your Own Gym** by Mark Lauren – A guide to bodyweight training.

- **The Whole30** by Melissa Hartwig Urban – A reset for healthy eating habits.
- **Strength Training Anatomy** by Frederic Delavier – Visual explanations of exercises.

Websites

- **ACE Fitness** (acefitness.org): Science-backed exercise and health tips.
- **Precision Nutrition** (precisionnutrition.com): Expert advice on eating for fitness.
- **Yoga with Adriene** (yogawithadriene.com): Free yoga videos for all levels.

Apps

- **Nike Training Club**: Guided workouts for different goals and levels.
- **Headspace**: Meditation and mindfulness for stress management.
- **FitOn**: Free fitness classes ranging from HIIT to Pilates.

Appendix D: Glossary of Fitness Terms

1. **Cardiovascular Exercise**: Activities that increase your heart rate, such as running, swimming, or cycling. Also known as cardio.

2. **Compound Movements**: Exercises that involve multiple muscle groups, such as squats, deadlifts, and push-ups.

3. **HIIT (High-Intensity Interval Training)**: A training technique involving short bursts of intense activity followed by brief recovery periods.

4. **Macronutrients**: Nutrients needed in large amounts: carbohydrates, proteins, and fats.

5. **Micronutrients**: Essential vitamins and minerals required in smaller amounts for health.

6. **Recovery**: Activities and rest are designed to allow the body to repair and grow stronger after exercise.

7. **Resistance Training**: Exercises designed to improve strength and endurance by working against resistance, such as weights or resistance bands.

8. **Resting Heart Rate**: The number of times your heart beats per minute while at rest, often used to gauge fitness levels.

9. **Static Stretching**: Stretching a muscle to its farthest point and holding the position, often used post-workout to enhance flexibility.

10. **Warm-Up**: This light activity is designed to prepare your body for more intense exercise by increasing blood flow and loosening muscles.

These appendices are designed to give you practical tools and foundational knowledge to take action. Use them to kickstart your fitness journey, adapt as needed, and keep learning along the way!